FINDING GOOD

One Family's Story of True Love in the Face of Cancer,
Celebrating Life's Blessings, and Spreading Positivity
as #TeamStone

**Johnathon Stone
and Sarah Stone**

For information contact: johnathon.stone@teamstonefindinggood.com

Cover design by Cara Baker, CMBakerDesign.com
Interior design by Amber Hargett
Backyard hammock photo on cover © Hayne Palmour Iv/San Diego
Union-Tribune via ZUMA Wire

ISBN: 978-0-692-10330-2

ADVANCE PRAISE
FOR FINDING GOOD

"If you are able to soak up 10% of the passion that this man has to share you will experience a new understanding of love and purpose in all that you do."

- Jairek Robbins,
bestselling author and performance coach

"Johnny's story is inspiring because it's real and told from the heart. His life is a living example of the idea that it's not what happens to you in life that counts, it's what you DO with what happens to you that counts. When life handed Johnny lemons, he made lemonade. Reading his book has inspired me to live with more gratitude and work harder to help others. It will do the same for you. A must read."

- Guy Spier,
investor and author of The Education of a Value Investor

"Riveting. Heartwarming. Inspiring. A story the strikes a chord with your soul."

- Cherilyn Jones,
intuitive coach

DEDICATION

*I'd like to give a special thank you to Lori Stone, Mary Shofner,
the crew of the USS ESSEX, the staff at UCSD Moore's Cancer Center,
"The Village" and Wendy Maze.*

*Most importantly, this book is for all the men and women who have had
or are currently battling cancer or hardship in life.*

- Johnathon Stone

FOREWORD

I was one of Sarah's nurses in her final days, and I consider that experience one of the greatest gifts I've ever received. In the short time we spent together, she touched me so deeply... she changed my life. Through this book, she can change yours as well.

I served in the United States military and then worked as a broadcast journalist; both roles offered me endless opportunities to meet new and incredibly inspiring people from all around the world. They gave me strength and grit, curiosity and compassion, and the ability to remain clearheaded and articulate under pressure.

So, when I decided to become a Critical Care nurse, I felt prepared. Fresh out of nursing school, marching into the world of Intensive Care, I was full of energy, eager to devour knowledge, ready to attack disease and save lives.

A wise mentor soon steered my career toward palliative care in the ICU, and I soon discovered that "winning" and "defeating" are different when it comes to battling cancer.

I didn't know Sarah Stone for long, but in our first hour together, I could see that this was not someone to be babied, pampered, or mollycoddled. There was a quiet power behind her eyes. She had grace and dignity, strength and complexity. She was authentic. And, she kept smiling! She insisted on taking selfies and made it clear that, above all else, her room was to be filled with peace and joy.

One of the greatest pleasures of nursing is getting to know a person's life story, connecting with them and making time for reminiscing. At Sarah's bedside, I heard a life story unlike any I'd ever heard before... a sweet teen romance that blossomed into a deeply devoted partnership... long nights in the NICU with tiny twins who struggled to survive... months and months of waiting for her beloved husband to complete his military tours, hoping he would return to his family, safe and sound. She talked about her diagnosis and the day they cut her long, beautiful red hair. On her last day, we would set aside locks of that same strawberry blond hair for their children to keep forever. Every sentence tore at my heartstrings. Although I kept my composure, my heart wept for her, and him, and their children and loved ones. I kept thinking, *This isn't fair!*

And yet, through it all, she smiled. That tiny, mighty redhead refused to let her spirit be overshadowed by struggles and tragedy. She insisted on seeing the beauty and opportunity in every challenge, every change, every moment. She insisted on joy. She embodied courage, acceptance, and surrender... and a bright, full-hearted vision for the future.

Navigating end of life care is intense and deeply challenging... and, it is a sacred privilege.

When a terminal patient's final moments come, the greatest service a nurse can provide is to make those moments just as beautiful as when a soul first enters this world. We strive to comfort to our patient and their family and, above all else, honor the patient's wishes (if they were able to express them in advance).

So many times, I've held the hand of a family member who insisted, "She's been sicker than this and come through so many times. She's a fighter! She's going to beat this!" Even though we both knew... this time, their loved one, my patient, would not pull through.

It's all too easy to get trapped in this snapshot of a family's tragedy. Many of my medical teammates (doctors, respiratory therapists, aides, and social workers), and our family and friends carry the heartache and loss of these moments for years, wondering what we could have done better. We struggle to accept that there comes a time when the physical body cannot do what our mind and spirit, family and medical team insist it can do. It can be so hard to let go... and to face what lies ahead.

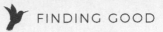

The truth is, all we have to do is stay present and make the most of this moment. That's all.

The love story of Johnathon and Sarah is incomparable to any you may have heard. Her resilience lives on like a song, through him, his children and their joy in finding the good in every day. After reading this life-changing book, it will live on through you, too.

I'll stop here and let him share their personal fairy tale – and the beautiful chapters that stretch into the joyful future she envisioned.

- Bridgette Lowe

TABLE OF CONTENTS

CHAPTER ONE

Love is not about how many days, months, or years you've been together. Love is about how much you love each other every day.

It's October 29th, 2016 in San Diego, California and my neighborhood community is getting ready for our annual Halloween party. My three daughters, Alyssa and Allie (nine-year-old twins) and Maddie (seven years old), run in and out of the master bedroom, putting on a fashion show for my wife, Sarah, with their costumes. Twirling beside the bed and giving their best poses, they then pause as Sarah reaches out from the bed and touches their costumes. Our youngest child, Jackson, plays on the floor.

"Make sure you bring home extra candy for me," she says, smiling from her pillow. Even though she is battling stage four appendix cancer, she finds something good to focus on. "I love you." The girls each kiss her before running out to put on their shoes.

"I won't be gone too long," I tell her, standing in the doorway with our adopted son, Jackson, in my arms. "My mom's right out here in the living room in case you need her."

"You go have fun," Sarah says. "Tell everyone I'll be there next time." I could tell she is disappointed that she's missing one of the cul-de-sac's holiday parties. Our neighborhood, known as "The Village," is tight-knit and sociable; on any given evening, we sit out in the street with lawn chairs and watch the kids throw water balloons or ride bikes. We are lucky to have neighbors who feel like family and who love our kids like their own. Lately though, Sarah hasn't been feeling well and my mom flew in to help us care for the kids.

Yesterday, Sarah was unable to travel to her doctor's appointment, so I went in her place to talk to her doctor. Her cancer is wearing her down physically; she is sick constantly and can't breathe well. At this point, after ten and a half months of battling cancer, she has a bad cough, is throwing up, and is now unable to do much without direct assistance. Her medication causes her to have hallucinations, which I try to keep the kids away from seeing so they aren't scared.

During the Halloween party, I get a phone call from her primary oncologist, a world-renowned doctor, requesting me to bring her into the hospital immediately.

"I just got her test results back," he says. "I'm on call tonight, so let's get her in now so I can focus on her."

The news hits me in the gut like a sucker punch. Trying my best to fight back tears, I motion to the girls to come over to me. The three of them run over, plastic pumpkin buckets filled and big smiles on their faces.

"I have to take mommy to the hospital. Whitney, Lindsay, Tasha, and Jenn are going to stay with you. Promise Daddy that you'll have fun and behave, okay?"

"Okay," they say and run back to play with their friends. My neighbors are always ready to help out whenever I need to take Sarah to the doctor, and I don't know where I'd be without their love, support, and homemade meals when I'm unable to cook.

I rush home to get Sarah. "We have to go in tonight so that they can help you," I say. I pack up her portable oxygen and her wheelchair and take her to the UC San Diego Health's Moore's Cancer Center in La Jolla, one of the top oncology programs in the nation. Whenever we go there, the team of nurses and doctors always make us feel as comfortable as possible.

They admit her and start giving her fluids and nutrients because she has

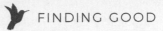

lost so much weight. The next twenty-four hours are tough. Sarah's coughing persists and I hold her hand, checking her every few minutes to make sure she is okay. The palliative team mentions at-home nurses and hospice, but even then, I don't realize that we are in the final days of Sarah's life.

"Are you okay, Johnny?" Sarah says, calling me by my nickname. "Do you have everything you need?" This is what I love about Sarah—she is always looking out for others, even when she is suffering. At this point, she can barely talk, but still looks out for me.

We wait patiently until her oncologist and medical team come in to discuss chemo and their plans for future treatment. In typical Sarah fashion, she smiles and tries to lighten the mood, even though she is weak.

"I bet the Cubs win the World Series," she says with a smile. We all laugh and the oncologist begins discussing chemo plans. After he leaves, she touches the nurse's arm. "I need a brownie and a glass of milk because I want a date with and my husband tonight," Sarah says. The nurse brings her a double chocolate brownie within minutes.

"Just like old times," I say, kissing her gently on her forehead. Sarah and I always loved to eat homemade brownies. After long days at work in the Navy as a Chief Petty Officer, I treasured my time at home having dinner with Sarah and the kids.

Sarah can only have a nibble and has me finish the rest, but I know she enjoys the chocolate. Despite everything going on, we still smile find the good at the beginning and end of each day. It is really hard sometimes, but we stick to that promise no matter what. We are a true team—Team Stone.

After the brownie, we talk about the future. I think Sarah knows that death is coming very soon, as much as I don't want to accept it.

"Promise me that, no matter what happens, you will continue to do good things, take good care of the kids and always be patient with them."

"You know I will." I squeeze her hand. She squeezes back.

"I'm always going to look out for you, even when I'm in Heaven. And you have to smile—find the good. Remember our promise."

"Every day," I say. "The kids and I will find the good always."

"I want you to also promise me that you'll move on...that you'll let yourself find someone to fall in love with. I want you to remarry."

"No, I don't want to think about that." I lean over in my chair and rest my head on the side of her bed. She brushes my hair with her fingertips, slowly, because she is weak.

"Johnny, yes. You deserve to be loved and to have someone loved by you."

We talk about the first time we fell in love and how crazy it is that life worked out for us. I crack a joke; she manages to laugh in between labored breaths. Soon she begins coughing again and one of her favorite nurses comes in to check in her.

"Johnny, are you heading to the cafeteria for any dinner? I will keep an eye on her if you are," the nurse offers.

"I'm good for now, but thank you. I appreciate it."

The nurse gives an encouraging smile to Sarah and closes the door again. Sarah is friends with everyone and all the nurses love her. The cafeteria staff know me well because I always go down there to grab a quick meal when I stay with her, and I'll talk to just about anyone. I love meeting new people, especially at the hospital. Tonight, I don't want to leave Sarah's side.

She looks at me, weak, but still manages a twinkle in her eyes.

"You are the love of my life. I have lived the exact life I have always dreamed of." We both know that true love does exist in the world, despite the hard things that happen. "Promise me that you'll move on with your life. You are meant to be a husband and a lover to someone else."

"I will, I promise. I don't want to think about that right now though." I kiss her hand and smile. "Get some sleep, okay? I'll be right here."

Around 2 a.m., Sarah's monitors start beeping and flashing like crazy. I jolt awake from my hospital recliner and watch as she struggles to get enough oxygen.

"Johnny," she cries out, her voice barely above a whisper. I grab the emergency call button and start pressing it as many times as my thumb will

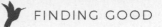

go. A handful of nurses come rushing in, followed by the on-call doctor.

"Something's wrong," I say, feeling panic rise in my chest. I back away from the bed as they try to drain fluid from her lungs with big needles and do everything they can to bring her breathing back to normal.

What's happening?

Two doctors take me aside and lower their voices so she can't hear.

"Listen, we have some bad news," the first doctor says. "You have about five minutes to decide. You have an extremely difficult choice now; you can put her on life support, and she'll suffer because she's in bad shape. We can't adequately treat a cancer patient on life support. Or, we can take her upstairs to the ICU and put her on oxygen and she'll have anywhere from four to forty-eight hours to live. I need you to decide now—we have to move quickly."

What do I do? How do I make the right choice? How do I find something good to hold on to? I am freaking out. Everything is happening too fast but at the same time, I feel like I'm in a nightmare.

"Please help me," I say as my voice cracks and I break down in front of the doctors. "I don't know what to do." Machines are beeping rapidly as if to signal that the end is coming. The nurses begin to cry with me. In this moment, I realize how much my wife is loved by everyone around her—and how life is never going to be the same.

I turn to Sarah and look her through my tears. She is half sedated and she winks, like she is telling me it is ok. She is ready to leave.

I now know what to do.

"Take her upstairs. Don't put her on life support. I just want to make her comfortable."

"You should bring the children to say goodbye," the second doctors says, touching my shoulder. The nurses immediately prepare to wheel her out of the room.

I sit down in a chair to call my mom, staring at the floor while the I wait for her to answer. It's the longest moment in my life. She picks up on the third ring.

"Mom, she's not going to make it. I need you to bring the kids as soon as you can."

When the kids arrive, they color pictures for Sarah and show them to her while she is still conscious in bed. They think this is like any other time when Sarah isn't feeling well. Our daughters are natural helpers and always want to cheer people up. At one point, I gather them around me to break the news to them, crayons still held in their little hands.

"Listen, this is the last time you'll see Mommy," I say, trying to hold myself together. "She is going to heaven soon and it's not your fault."

Don't lose it. You need to be strong for them, I think to myself. I take a deep breath and focus. *It's my turn to step up. If we are all going to melt down, the family will be lost. I have to be their anchor.*

"Daddy is okay. I'm here for you and I never want you to worry." They don't fully understand what is going on. "Mommy is going to be leaving us soon and this is going to be the last time you're going to see her." The twins are quiet and Maddie puts her head on my shoulder.

The nurses are standing at the edge of the room crying. I am crying too, now, despite my best efforts to be strong and positive. Sarah's father and brother arrive that night from Illinois, but her mother is unable to travel because she is battling stage four breast cancer. It's an unthinkable situation that everyone tries to process. Sarah is able to make one final phone call to say goodbye.

"It's okay, Mom," She says, as I listen to her speak slowly. Each breath counts. Every word is important. They are very close and her mother always thought she'd pass before her daughter, even with cancer. Her mother asks why this is happening.

"Because it's meant to be," Sarah softly replies. "Mom, it's okay," she repeats. You will all be okay."

Our neighborhood friends from "The Village" arrive as well. One by one, Sarah finds the strength to give a "pass down," or words of wisdom, to each

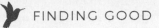

of them. She doesn't want them to mourn her death and instead tells them to celebrate her.

Her father and brother arrive five hours later and rush from San Diego International Airport, racing time to have a goodbye.

"I want you to try and do your best," Sarah says to her brother. "Love your family. I know things are going to be hard, but I want you to try for me."

Everyone trickles out, except for me and the kids. The image of our daughters and son kissing their mother one final time is something I can never forget. The nurses look at each other to try and pull themselves together. They manage smiles for the kids. The team at UC San Diego Moores has been like a second family to us and this is tough for them, too.

Finally, the room clears and it is just the two of us.

"Johnny, I wrote a letter for you," she says. It's in our nightstand. "I want you to read it when you go home. It's going to make everything better."

"No way," I reply. "How will it make everything better? You are my best friend. You are all I've known. How am I going to go on?" I am losing my mind. In that moment, I am struggling to find the good. But, at least she is able to talk.

"Johnny, do good things after I am gone," she says. I wipe tears from my face and she begins to cry, too. After a moment of silence, she asks, "Do you think people will forget me?"

I begin sobbing and kiss her hand. "No, never Sarah, do you realize how many lives you've impacted?"

She smiles, but I see the color draining from her face. Her normally rosy cheeks have paled and her body is fragile and stiff.

I look her straight in the eyes and say, "It will be my mission to keep your legacy alive. You've changed the world for the better."

Her last spoken words to me are, "I have zero regrets in my life and that's because of you."

I hold Sarah's hand through the entire night and never let go. I watch her drift in and out of sleep. I am afraid that she will pass before I can say goodbye. She previously said wanted to go after Halloween so she doesn't ruin it for the kids moving forward. As every hour ticks by on my watch I am constantly touching her chest to make sure her precious heart is still beating.

When the morning of November 1st, 2016 breaks, the nurse checks her vitals. It is the same nurse from the day before and she has specifically requested to be with Sarah as she passes.

"It's only going to be a few more minutes. She doesn't have much longer," she says.

What am I going to do? Nothing prepares you for the moment you lose the love of your life.

"If you want to climb into bed and hold her, it's okay. She can't talk anymore, but she can write to you."

I climb into bed with a pen and pad of paper and wrap my arms around her, trying to keep myself composed. The final moments are surreal. So many moments when I've held my wife and now this was the last time. I point to the paper in her lap. She barely moves the pen across the pad to write a final message:

Big Gulps in heaven?

"Seriously?" I say. Even in her final moments, Sarah had a sense of humor. Whenever it was a hot day, she would sit outside and I'd bring her a Big Gulp from 7-Eleven—her favorite treat. When she got sick, she was unable to drink soda and we'd joke about Big Gulps. "Yes, you are going to sit up in Heaven and drink all the Big Gulps you want." She winks at me again; her breathing slows.

"It's going to be okay, I will always, always love you," I whisper in her ear. I look in her eyes as she takes her very last breath.

Then, she's gone. Sarah Kay Stone is only 29.

I cry for what feels like a lifetime. *God, why is this happening? The love of my life is gone! The mother of my four children is gone. How am I going to be a single dad?* I wonder how my life is going to change when I leave this room, this hospital that has become a second home over the last year.

Sarah's father and brother follow me back to the van as I push an empty wheelchair. We go home to try and break the news to the kids.

How am I going to do this? I don't know anything about raising girls and Jackson has special needs... What am I going to do?

When I enter my home, it's full of memories. Sarah's presence is everywhere. I can hear Sarah's voice in my mind, as if she is right there with me:

"Johnny, you have to be strong for the kids. It's game time. Go take care of business. You have to keep moving forward."

I gather the girls and Jackson in our back room. "Mommy has gone to heaven," I say. We all cry together and I stay there, hugging them for as long as they need. The best mother in the world is gone and I'm not sure what to do next. In this moment, my children are my good.

I realize that I quickly need to make funeral arrangements, but I have never been to a funeral. Now I had to plan one for the love of my life.

The letter... Sarah left me a letter.

That night, I muster up the courage to go to the nightstand in the master bedroom. Inside the drawer, I find a letter in a small, white envelope.

FROM SARAH:
I want my life celebrated, not mourned.
No black clothes for immediate family.
I'd like someone who knew me well to speak about my life.

I want it emphasized that I loved life and was passionate
about my children. That I loved fiercely and was blessed
to have married my best friend at such a young age.

Sarah includes detailed instructions on how to plan the funeral, how she wants her service, what to dress her in, what songs to play, and how she wants her headstone to look.

In this moment, I feel less alone. God won't fail me and neither will Sarah. The kids and I will keep going, finding the good that Sarah loved in each day.

It's time to keep my promise. Sarah's legacy will live on. I will find the good in each day with my kids and share it with the world.

CHAPTER TWO

There is good in everything.

I t was 2003 when I first met Sarah. My parents raised me to work hard growing up, and I spent countless days out in the farm fields of Clinton, Illinois bailing hay and helping with chores. I kept to myself for the most part, until one day when I learned that there were some kids my age who lived about two miles from me. I decided to ride my dirt bike over.

I was always good at talking to people and making new friends, so I introduced myself to a few people, including a younger boy named Kalan, who became my best friend. Kalan was dating (which wasn't real dating at that age) a girl named Heather, who was best friends with Sarah. At the time, Sarah was mysterious; I heard a lot about her through various conversations with people but didn't know what she looked like. This was back in the time of AOL Instant Messenger and people were connected online but never talked in person. Living in a rural area with homes sometimes miles apart made it hard to socialize unless someone had a car.

Eventually, when I got my license, I was at Sunset Inn and Suites, the only nice hotel in town at the time. It had an indoor pool and sauna and you could swim as long as you wanted for just five dollars. Kalan and I always went there every Friday night because we didn't have a ton of money but wanted to socialize. I remember signing in at the front desk with Kalan and talking to the manager when a voice chimed in from behind.

"Hey guys!" Heather said, walking in with a backpack and towel over her arm. A short, fiery redhead with long, curly hair was beside her. She didn't even really look at me. I nudged Kalan.

"Who is that?" I said, staring at but trying to not seem obvious. Kalan nudged me back and smiled.

"That's Sarah," he replied. I watched them walk past and Sarah ignored me. I was more curious than ever.

The pool area was buzzing with teens playing music, laughing, and doing cannonballs into the pool, which was against the rules. As our group of friends chatted, Sarah and I realized that we actually didn't like each other. In fact, we almost couldn't stand each other! We were the same person with a take charge, get-business-done type of personality. She was sarcastic with a smart mouth, just like me as a teen.

I got along with her friends, however, and continued to show up at the pool every Friday. Like clockwork, Sarah was there with her friends as well, but we didn't interact much. Eventually, Sarah started having movie nights at her house. She conveniently planned them around when she knew I would be working at a place called The Shack, a classic, all-American diner that served up burgers and shakes. While I was putting in extra hours to make quick cash, all my friends were at Sarah's movie nights.

One day in 2004, before I graduated high school, Sarah had another movie night (which I wasn't invited to) and Kalan ended up leaving his cell phone there.

"Hey, can you do me a favor and drop by and get it from her?" he asked.

"No way, are you kidding?" I said.

"Come on man, it will take like two seconds." So, I stopped by without calling ahead of time. I knocked and Sarah answered the door.

"What are you doing here?"

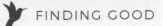

"I'm just here to get Kalan's phone. He said he forgot it."

Sarah had three adopted sisters that were playing in the living room. We walked in and her parents gave me weird looks from the kitchen because I was an older boy in the house. I immediately tried to help Sarah look for the phone, so I could get out of there as fast as possible. We started to chat as we turned over couch cushions and I realized we had more positive qualities in common than we thought. We found the good in each other.

"Well, thanks for helping me find his phone," I said, as we stood at her front door.

"No problem. See you around," she said.

We made eye contact and I felt an electric jolt and I knew that she felt it, too.

Whoa, I think I like this girl.

I had a big, red 1978 Mercury Marquis that I had bought for $500 called Clifford.

"Is that your car?" she asked, laughing. We talked for half an hour more and the conversation flowed and was great.

"How'd it go?" Kalan asked with a smirk later when I dropped off his phone.

"Actually, not so bad. I think I have a crush on her," I said.

I connected to dial-up Internet, logged into MSN Messenger and saw that she was online. We started talking more and more.

One night, my friends and I were supposed to go swimming, but no one could go. I called Sarah to see if she wanted to go. After a few rings, Sarah's dad answered the phone.

"Hi, is Sarah there?"

"No, she isn't." *Click.* Sarah's dad hung up on me! After ten minutes, I tried again, palms sweating, because I never give up easily on something I really want. Sarah ended up answering, but her parents wouldn't let her go swimming. We talked for about two hours. By this point, we were good friends.

Every day when I got out from high school early to do a work study program, I would go home and email Sarah. We went to different high schools, so the Internet or phone were the most common ways of our communication. We would send each other long emails each day—her from study hall at her school. We told each other everything about ourselves through daily emails for an entire year. When things got tough, I was always there to encourage her.

You're amazing. It's going to be okay, I promise, I would write.

By this point, I had signed up for the Navy and was leaving at the end of the summer after graduation.

When I graduated in May of 2004, out of all the girls in the group of friends. Sarah and her friend Brandi were the only two to come congratulate me. They followed me back to my house for a graduation party with my family.

"Congrats, Johnny!" Sarah said, and gave me a hug. She left later that night to go study with another guy that I didn't like. I felt my first pangs of jealousy. After the sun dipped down over the horizon, a message popped up on my AOL Instant Messenger.

I wish you could come hang out, she wrote.

During the beginning of summer, Sarah had a campout at her house. Kalan and I were supposed to rough it outside in my raggedy tent away from the girls, who were going to stay in the convenience of the living room. Kalan ended up not being able to go, so I was stuck outside alone. I remember laying in the tent during the middle of the night when a big thunderstorm rolled in, soaking me. I was forced to come inside to sleep. The funny part about it is that Sarah was trying to set me up with Brandi, who eventually dozed off on the couch. Sarah and I sat on the floor, talking and laughing.

One of the first fundraising experiences we attended together was a local Relay for Life event for the American Cancer Society. Sarah and I were the only ones to attend out of our group of friends. A song came on the radio and I grabbed her hand and pretended to sing to her. I didn't let go. I was

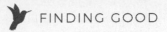

so nervous now to be around her because the energy was building. When we looked up at each other, we knew something special was happening. We were finally a couple, but were too shy to admit it.

That summer, we wrote it journals: mine was black, hers was pink, and we loved to write back and forth in each other's. We called them the "Johnny and Sarah" books. Every week, we exchanged them frequently to read what the other had written. One day when Sarah and I were alone in her living room, talking about the Johnny and Sarah books, we shared our first kiss. It was one of the most amazing moments in my entire life. It was magical and lasted a few minutes.

I'm going to marry this girl, I thought to myself.

I was leaving for the Navy and she still had a year of high school left. We didn't call each other boyfriend/girlfriend for a while, but I told her, "I know we're going to end up together, I can just feel it." She eventually came to me with her Sarah book and asked me to read it. She left the room while I read the words: *Johnny Stone, I'm in love with you and never want to be apart from you. I'm scared and don't want to lose you.*

I had written the same in my book.

"Come here," I called to her. I handed her my Johnny book. "I have something in my book, too. Read this." I watched as her eyes lit up when she read my words to her. We hugged and cried together as we thought about the few months left before I had to report for duty.

I got a temporary job at a factory in order to make enough money to take her on dates. However, Sarah was the one who had to drive because I had gotten in trouble for speeding. We found the good in it though; I taught her to drive a stick. I spent a lot of time with her family as well, and they saw that I was trying to be responsible and treated their daughter with love and respect. They grew to like me after some time.

One of Sarah's sisters would watch the door at her house so we could make out. She would and alert us when her parents were back so we didn't get busted. Every day after a long day of work, I would head straight for Sarah's house. I was even allowed to stay over at Sarah's house in the guest room beside her room. We'd lie awake late at night, communicating through knocks on the shared wall. Our code was: three times for "I love you," four times for "I love you too," two times for "I want a kiss."

My parents were annoyed that I was spending so much time away from the family, especially since I was leaving for the Navy soon. But Sarah and I wanted to make every moment count. Soon, I quit my job at the factory so I could spend more time at Sarah's. When my mom found out, she drove over to Sarah's house and made me go home. I was grounded, so Sarah got me a box of Fruity Pebbles (the cereal I would always eat at her house) and I carried around her Sarah book as I moped. Then, my parents made me go on a nine-day trail ride even though I was against it. While on the trail, I spent as much time as I could at a pay phone that I got up and walked to every morning before breakfast. Sometimes, it poured rain outside. My friends on the trip thought I was nuts, but I couldn't stand to be away from her.

"Is there any way I can go home?" I asked my mom, who was still annoyed but caved at the sight of young love. There was another woman on the trip who was heading home five days early.

"Just catch a ride with her," Mom said.

When I arrived home, Sarah was waiting for me. We'd rent DVDs from Family Video and try to snuggle on the couch. "Hand check," her mom would say from time to time. We had a special spot we'd go to talk—in the woods behind her house. We carved a heart and our initials into a special tree. It's still there today. So many people tried to convince her to break up with me, saying that it wouldn't last and that we were young and foolish to want to make such a serious commitment so fast. But, we knew we were meant to be together. I knew Sarah had to be my wife and we needed to create a life together.

I left for Navy in January of 2005. It was the second saddest day of my life. I cried during the entire two hour drive to Chicago.

"It's only boot camp," the recruiter said. "You'll be back soon."

I was one of the only people who had letters to read every single Sunday when mail was distributed. We were only allowed to read and write letters

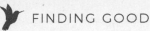

once a week, always on Sunday. On a weeknight during boot camp, I reopened a letter Sarah had previously sent without realizing she had stuffed red confetti in the shape of lips in the bottom of the envelope. I was covered as I lay in my bunk bed—this stuff was everywhere. Fearing punishment, I quietly hopped down while the rest of the guys were asleep and spent an hour picking up confetti off the floor with my bare hands.

Sarah was my everything and we counted the days until we could see each other. I graduated boot camp in March of 2005 and went to Pensacola, Florida for A-School. My mother and aunt brought Sarah down a few times when they came. She was still a senior in high school at the time.

I took Sarah for a walk on the beach. I had set up a monthly payment plan on an engagement ring that pretty much tapped out my E-1 salary, but I knew I had to propose. I took her to an old bench by the water where we liked to sit and talk.

"Hey, what's that?" I said, pointing behind her. She looked away and I bent down on one knee and quickly pulled out the ring.

"Sarah, will you marry me?"

We started crying and she said yes. She went back to Illinois as my fiancée and started waitressing at a place called Ted's Garage. We made very little money, but I promised her that she would have her dream wedding. We saved and saved. I lived off ramen noodles and macaroni and cheese. After several months, we paid for everything on our own.

I moved to San Diego to my first duty station. A few months later, I flew home and we had our dream wedding.

True love exists and at that moment, we knew we had we made it.

CHAPTER THREE

With love, nothing is impossible.

I remember slow dancing at our wedding reception and whispering into Sarah's ear, "We did it." A lot of people say marriage is just a piece of paper, but to us it was a bond—through sickness and health. We went to the Sunset Inn where it all began. Sarah and I had made a promise to wait until marriage to be intimate and our first night together was special. Some couples have friendship without passion or passion without friendship; Sarah and I had both.

My best man, Jason, who was stationed with me in San Diego came over later with Sarah's sister, Cassie, to hang out and eat pizza. We spent two days together at the Inn before loading up Sarah's little 2005 Nissan Sentra with all of her stuff and driving to San Diego.

We gassed up and left with nothing but love. I had a little apartment waiting for us in Imperial Beach. At the time, Imperial Beach wasn't the best area to live in, but I had two jobs and was trying to get by. We were pumped and ready to get our life started together. We were two small town kids with nothing but love and a big dream of making it in California.

When we arrived, we had an air mattress, some pots and pans, and some gift certificates. We went to Walmart and got some cleaning supplies and food items. Back then, air mattresses didn't come with a pump, so it took me an hour and a half to blow it up by mouth. I was sitting there blowing, looking at Sarah as she laughed at me. She stepped on the mattress to blow air back in my face. We had a quilt that her grandmother had made and a few cheap pillows. Life was simple, but we were grateful. We had each other, and that's all we needed.

I was an E-2 and had to get up at 4 a.m. and didn't want to leave her. I loved her so much and didn't want to be apart. Every single morning, the air mattress had gone flat and I would kiss Sarah goodbye, thank her for everything she did at home, and take our one car to work. I'd come home and we didn't have money to do anything, so we'd find free ways to make memories. One of our favorite things was to go see movies on the base or at a cheap drive-in down the street.

The laundry room at our apartment required us to put money on a card. Sometimes we didn't have enough money to put on the card to dry the clothes and we had to hand wash and hang our clothes outside on the back fence. I knew I wanted to do something better for Sarah and I vowed to do better. I looked out the sliding glass door at the laundry.

"I am 100% happy, Johnny: this is life. I don't need anything special." Sarah said and wrapped her arms around me in a hug.

How am I going to do this? I thought. I felt like a failure. I didn't want to go back home and live in a trailer.

Day by day, we lived life. We had talked about kids and knew we wanted them. Sarah wasn't on birth control and we wanted to allow God to bring children when it was his time.

We were pretty "boring" – we had never smoked a cigarette, got arrested, or did anything scandalous like some of our peers growing up. We were ornery but never got in big trouble. The only bad thing that happened was me getting two speeding tickets that previous summer.

One day when I came home, Sarah said she had missed her monthly cycle. I had no experience with kids—diapers, bottles, anything! We went to the

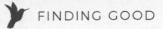

99 cent store to get a pregnancy test. I spent five dollars on tests just to be sure. I watched Sarah as she took the tests, one by one...and one by one, each test was positive!

Team Stone was official.

We had a two-bedroom apartment and Sarah was excited to decorate.

"Johnny, it's definitely a girl!"

"No way, it has to be a boy," I replied.

She paused and looked around the apartment and started to cry. "How are we going to afford all this?"

"That's where I come in. You don't need to worry. I will not let us fail. I will make this happen." And I was determined to follow through on that promise to her. I refused to let her and our baby down.

A few days later, I applied for a second job at the rec center on the base.

"Look, I'm just an E-2 with a kid on the way," I said to the manager. "I need to make sure I make enough money and am able to support my wife and kid. I'll work whatever hours you need. Once I'm done with my mechanic shift, I'm yours each day."

They hired me on the spot. I was working my Navy job and putting another forty hours a week at the rec center maintaining the mini golf course, cleaning the batting cages, taking the coins out, dealing poker to junior sailors, and selling food. The great thing about the rec center job was that I could bring Sarah along and not sacrifice my time with her. I would work behind the counter and Sarah would sit on a small couch in the front of the counter and eat snacks. We saved our money and counted our blessings.

One night, as I was wiping down the counter at the end of the night, Sarah said, "I think I am going to have twins." I laughed and didn't believe her, but She was convinced that it would be twins. She even told her mom and friends. After a few weeks, she called me at work during the day, which she never did. When my coworker handed over the receiver, I felt scared. scared when I picked up the phone, my hands greasy from changing out an engine.

"Johnny! I was right!" she said with excitement.

"About what, honey? Are you okay?"

"We're having twins!"

"Holy cow...are you serious?"

I stood there, dirty and sweaty, feeling stunned. I was having TWINS. When I didn't say anything for a moment, she reassured me.

"I know you're freaking out, Johnny, but we've got this."

I knew she was right. We had enough love to power the entire planet, so we would navigate twins like every other situation, positive and always finding gratitude.

"Alright, "I said. "It's game time."

When I came home one day from work, Sarah had a teddy bear and a pack of diapers waiting on the kitchen table.

"You're going to learn how to change a diaper today," she said with a smile. I had been worried that I wouldn't be able to change diapers and she could tell that it was bothering me. So, she took the teddy bear and diapered it in about five seconds. "Now, it's your turn. Don't be shy," she said, handing me a diaper. She patiently watched as I fumbled through one failed attempt after another.

"I'm never going to get the hand of this," I said.

"Yes, you are. Do it again," she would say, "You've got this, Johnny." I felt like I was in the *Karate Kid* but I got to the point where I could do it with my eyes closed. (Not that I actually would.) Then, she started teaching me everything she knew about babies. Sarah's motherly instincts were epic.

At an ultrasound appointment, the doctor announced, "Congratulations, you are having a boy, and we can't tell what the other one is yet."

A boy!

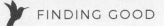

I was so excited but I could tell that Sarah was bummed. We went to Target that afternoon and I said, "Alright, we're going to get some baseball caps and tons of blue." We started getting a few things and I watched her walk around the baby clothes without saying much.

"I really wanted a girl. I thought it would be a girl. I hope the other one is a girl," she said, touching a pink lace baby dress.

At our next ultrasound appointment, the doctor informed us that they had made a mistake and we were in fact having TWO girls. I looked at Sarah with a smile. "You did this! You jinxed us." The look on her face was breathtaking. She was so happy, which made me happy. Our second Target trip was all pink.

Sarah was getting big and I was promoted to E-3 in the Navy. We went home to Illinois to visit when she was six months pregnant and her feet were swollen and hurting her. By then, we weren't on the air mattress. Thankfully, my salary allowed us to move into a three-bedroom house in Lemon Grove and a friend from work gave us a bed.

"Johnny," Sarah whispered one night. "I think I had an accident."

I woke up from a deep sleep to see her standing beside the bed looking at a wet spot on the mattress.

"Okay," I said, getting up quickly to help. "Hold on and I'll get a towel." When I came out of the bathroom, she gripped the side of the bed and cried out in pain. Right there, in front of me, I watched her water break. I had no clue what to do! Our bag wasn't packed, so I threw a few things together and rushed her to Balboa Hospital where she was evaluated.

"Mr. Stone, your wife needs a C-section right away. We're taking her back now," the doctor said. It made sense, because Sarah was 5'2" and having twins was too dangerous for her to have a normal delivery.

I had to change into hospital scrubs and wear a blue mask before I was allowed to go back into the operating room with her. It all went by so fast! She squeezed my hand, scared, and I remember them cutting her stomach.

"You've got this; I'm not going to leave you," I said.

Alyssa was pulled out first, at 1 pound 9 ounces, and I cut her umbilical cord. Fourty seconds later, Allison was pulled out at 2 pounds, 3 ounces. Two girls! They were rushed off before we could hold them. We were both scared because we didn't know what was going on.

"I want to see my babies as soon as possible," Sarah said, bringing out her feisty redhead side. I wheeled her down to the Neonatal Intensive Care Unit (NICU). They were tiny, jaundiced, and Allison ("Allie" as we nicknamed her) was having trouble breastfeeding from the start.

Alyssa always had pink on, Allie always had purple on. I could never tell the difference between the two until later when Alyssa developed a birthmark. But, Sarah always knew.

The babies spent three months in the NICU. I had to go back to work with the Navy. We still had only one car. The hardest thing was going home without our babies. They literally had to ask us to leave. This was the real beginning of us finding the good about everything.

Our daily routine was to get up at 4 a.m., I would drop Sarah off at the hospital to sit with the twins all day, I would go to work, go to the hospital and sit with Sarah until visiting hours ended for the evening. Finally, the hospital let us stay the night. Our first night was chaotic; when one baby would cry it would wake up the other. We were trying to feed them, change diapers.

We are in for it, I thought to myself.

The hospital finally cleared the twins for discharge. There we were, Team Stone, with a small car, two car seats in the back and heading home for good. It was game time!

I carried both girls, one baby in each arm and secured them in their carriers. Sarah sat in the back between them. I drove about 35 mph in the rush San Diego traffic, cars honking horns, but I wanted to make sure they were safe. "Hold on to them," I told Sarah.

When were home, that was it. We had to figure it out together. The twins

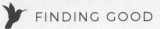

cried, we changed diapers, fed them, and tried to soothe them to sleep. We were young, we looked at each other we reassurance, and we lived each day. Whenever Sarah needed to get up with the babies in the middle of the night, I was right there with her.

After a long day at work, I would rush home and relieve Sarah of her duties so she could relax. She was so exhausted. I would watch her lay down on the bed and fall asleep. I'd be up at midnight and 3 am and then get ready for work at 4 a.m. For a while, it was challenging, but we always stayed positive. We quickly found our stride and decided it was time to add a third child to Team Stone.

When the twins were two years old, I was on a deployment and Sarah moved to Illinois temporarily so she could be with her family while she was pregnant with Madelyn. I was lucky enough to make it back in time for Maddie's birth. Only a few days after she was born, we packed all three kids into our car and drove straight home to California. It was a challenging 30-hour drive and we only stopped to take quick breaks, feed the twins, and nurse baby Maddie. When we rolled into San Diego, we moved into a new home and were excited to be a family of five.

CHAPTER FOUR

Family is more than just blood.

S arah had Factor V Leiden, a rare bleeding disorder that can cause an increase in blood clotting. Despite this disorder, we were lucky to be blessed with a third daughter, Maddie, two years after the twins were born, without major issues. Team Stone was a family of five and life was chaotic but blessed. During deployment, Sarah handled the three girls all on her own, but never complained.

It was too risky for her to carry a fourth child. We knew we wanted a boy to complete Team Stone, but adoption was out of the picture because it was too expensive. Growing up, Sarah had three foster sisters that were eventually adopted, so we decided to start the process of fostering. Angels Foster Family Network is a nonprofit in San Diego that ensures infants and children five and younger in foster care throughout San Diego County receive a loving home. During an info night, we learned all about their incredible mission and knew we were in the right place. We went to the very next training session.

"How long do you think it will take to find a child, Johnny? What if it doesn't work out?" Sarah said to me as we drove home from training.

"You have to have faith. This is all going to work out, you'll see," I said. They told us that it took about four to six months to get approved as a resource family, meaning we'd be eligible to foster a child. Sarah and I

29

remained committed to doing what it took to become certified. We decided to sign up to foster as many kids as possible until the right child came along for our family. Sarah and I had a lot of love to share. Sure enough, the day we received certification we also got a call about a child who needed us.

In April of 2013, I answered my phone while at a beach cleanup with Sarah and the kids—one of the things we liked to do as a family to promote good in our community. There was a two-day-old baby boy who was in critical need of a family. The social worker said we could pick him up the very next day!

"Sarah—you're never going to believe this," I said, with a big smile. "We've got a baby boy, his name is Dragen."

We didn't know anything about Dragen, so we were not sure what race or ethnicity he would be, but those things didn't matter to us. Sarah walked back first to see him and when she returned, she had the biggest smile on her face.

"Johnny, look! He has red hair just like the girls." She held up a pale, redheaded boy who looked exactly like he was one of us. We bonded with Dragen right away and loved him like our own.

After a few months, it was apparent that he had some developmental issues and special needs because he wasn't hitting his milestones like a child his age normally would. For instance, he wasn't rolling over when he should have. He had severe global delays and was on the autism spectrum, which meant that he would hit his milestones later in life. His mother had used drugs while pregnant, which impacted Dragen's development in the womb. But, it didn't matter to us. He felt like our son and fit right in with Team Stone. Everywhere we went, we went as a family. As each month passed we saw how the girls fell more and more in love with their little "brother," and Sarah and I were growing nervous that he would be adopted by a family.

The journey took a while and we weren't sure if we would be given the chance to adopt. Most foster situations are for adoption and the goal is to get the child back to their biological family. There was a chance he would be reunited with his birth mother, if she was able to get clean. To us, the guaranteed good in the situation was to give Dragen as much love and as

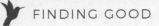

many positive experiences as we could during the time we had him. We were so blessed with three healthy girls and a beautiful baby boy, even if only for a little while. We knew God would take care of the rest.

By summer of 2015, Dragen's mother had passed on the street and died of a severe drug overdose. The best day of our lives as Team Stone was when we legally adopted Dragen, now renamed Jackson, and I got one month of leave to be with the family. Everything was going great.

I was promoted to an E-7 and later received orders that I needed to leave in a week, on a Sunday at 10 p.m., to fly out and meet a ship overseas. It definitely was a bummer but we tried to make the best of it and prepare for my time away. Deployments are never easy on any military family. You never know what will happen during a deployment, so you make the most of the time you have with your family. It was hard to leave the kids but I knew Sarah would help them get through the time apart. The night that I flew out, we pulled up to the airport together as a family in our mini-van. Everyone was crying.

I was worried about simple but important things: Jackson finally saying his first words, Maddie learning to ride her bike without training wheels, and playing dress up with the twins. All the memory-making moments you miss when you are in the military. But I was motivated to go out and serve my country as a brand-new chief.

Sarah's got it. She's an awesome military spouse, I thought to myself. It's true. Military spouses learn very quickly to be the mom and the dad, mechanic, plumber...whatever is necessary. Thankfully, it ended up being a smooth deployment for most of the time. We grew a lot as a family but never grew out of love. However, soon we faced our biggest challenge as Team Stone...

Near the final three weeks of deployment, I called Sarah to check in on the family. Previously, her mother had batted breast cancer and won; unfortunately, I learned that the breast cancer had returned and spread.

"Do you want me to fly home? I can get there if you need me," I said.

"I'm okay," Sarah said. "I just am having a hard time eating. My stomach hurts a lot. It could be stress."

"I don't want you dealing with this and taking care of the kids all by yourself," I replied. Sarah was like a superwoman when it came to parenting, but I could tell she wasn't feeling good. We always tried to balance the kids; when I was home I would let her sleep in on weekends and would take the kids out for ice cream or to play in the cul-de-sac with the neighbors. Sarah loved cooking and the fact that she didn't have an appetite made me concerned.

"No, you're so close to being done," she said. "Please, focus on your mission. You'll see us soon."

Since I had made chief that year, I was scheduled to be one of the first people off the ship when we pulled into port three weeks later. It was a huge homecoming. Tons of families waited with signs and balloons; news crews covered the event to film reunions between wives and children and sailors. There were thousands of us coming home.

I stood on deck and scanned the crowd; bright, handmade signs that said, "Welcome Home" were waving at the crew. I eventually spotted Sarah.

Something was very wrong.

She had lost so much weight, especially in her face, except her stomach was unusually large. It looked like she was pregnant, but she wasn't.

As I made my way off the ship, we embraced and she cried. "I've missed you so much."

My priority was to get her to the doctor that week. After a bunch of tests, they didn't know what was causing her symptoms. Disappointed and frustrated, we returned home. Two weeks later, she woke up in pain one morning and called out to me.

"Where does it hurt?" I asked, "How bad is it?" The kids and I were attempting to fix breakfast while singing their favorite Disney songs.

"Everywhere," she said, struggling to sit up in bed.

"I'll ask one of the neighbors to watch the kids while we go to the ER."

At the hospital, I watched as an ultrasound was performed on Sarah's stomach area. I'll never forget the look of concern that crossed the technician's face. A bunch of doctors quickly gathered in the room.

"We have some bad news for you. You have a tumor the size of a grapefruit on your ovary and a second beside your stomach. We will need to operate immediately," one said.

It was December 15th.

Tumor? How could this be real? I thought as Sarah gripped my hand. *What would I do with the kids?*

"Can we wait until after Christmas?" I asked.

"No, we'll have to move fast on this. We have to do prep tomorrow and surgery the next day."

Sarah and I looked at each other, stunned. She started to cry, which made me cry. Nothing can prepare you for a tumor. Was it cancer? Would it be okay? Her mother was already going through cancer and now Sarah was sick? My emotions were haywire; I knew that we had a choice in that moment: we could find the good or we could go in the deep hole of fear and lose faith. Our family depended on our faith. I had four kids now to think about.

"Johnny, we've got this," Sarah said.

"I know, it's just unexpected," I said, taking a deep breath to calm down.

"Promise me we'll find the good. Promise me we'll find a reason to smile every night before we go to bed."

"We always do," I replied. "I love you more than anything."

When I looked into her eyes, I knew this was about to be a hard, tough journey. If Sarah and I both focused on all the bad stuff, it would make whatever time we had left miserable. There was no point in that.

Two days later, Sarah was in surgery for almost right hours. The sun dipped below the horizon as the doctor finally came to me in the waiting room. "We got both tumors out; the operation was successful, but, I'm afraid

I have some bad news. we ended up having to do a full hysterectomy. It's not ovarian cancer like thought—it's appendix cancer, and it has spread. Appendix cancer is extremely rare; only one person in a million will develop it. We will need to discuss next steps..."

This was it; my worst nightmare was coming true.

"Let me tell her, please. If you break the news it will only discourage her. We're a team for a reason."

They led me to her hospital room where I sat waiting as she recovered. *What was I going to say? How do you tell someone they have cancer?*

The anesthesia wore off and Sarah winked at me. I took her hand in mine and rubbed it to keep her calm.

"They figured out what it was," I said. "The doctor came out and told me it's cancer. He said it's in your appendix... and it's spread."

Sarah looked at me, then away for a moment and was quiet. "Johnny, we've got this."

We never asked for a timeline or when they thought she would pass.

"I need to be out of here before Christmas," she told the on-duty nurse.

"The chances of that happening are slim; in order for you to be discharged, you will need to walk at least three laps around the floor." The nurse said. Sarah was determined. Eventually, she made her three laps and was allowed to go home—right in time for Christmas. Sarah always knew that the mind is so powerful; whenever we were up against something that scared us or seemed impossible, we reminded each other to find something to focus on to get us there. She was only focused on the kids and being there for them as they opened presents.

Sarah got in a wheelchair and we went back to "The Village." The kids were at a neighbor's house. I wheeled Sarah up to the front door and she rang the doorbell. When the girls saw her, they came running over with Jackson in tow. Team Stone was reunited.

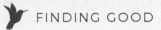

"Mommy! You got to come home for Christmas!" Allie said, beaming from ear to ear. It was the best Christmas we had ever had.

Fast forward about two weeks. Doctors found out the cancer spread to her bones. (I'm not going to lie; It was extremely difficult to find the good.) Now we were getting scared together. Sarah seemed more stressed with each check. Finally, they did the last check of the day—her brain. If things were bad there, we would be in trouble. Thankfully, it didn't appear in her brain.

That was our good. Even though it was stage four all over her body, her brain was okay. We spent several hours crying together, picking out fight songs, and trying to find things to laugh about. Team Stone needed to rally if we were going to make it through.

"We will need to start chemo immediately to prevent it from spreading more. Hopefully, we will be able to shrink the tumors. You may lose your hair; there's a 50/50 chance," a doctor said.

"Will I still be able to donate my hair?" Sarah asked immediately.

"No, once you begin chemo, you can't donate hair."

"All right," she said.

"Give me the hair clippers right now. I don't care, Johnny is going to cut my hair."

What? Wait a minute, I thought. I had never cut my wife's hair before... and now, she wanted me to shave her entire head. It was one of the hardest things to do.

"Someone out there is going through a tough time. They need this, Johnny." She sat up in her bed and began braiding her hair. I watched her hands shake from how weak her body was, but she was determined.

"Do you want me to help?", I asked.

"I've got it, but you need to cut it. I want to donate it right away."

I gently held her braid, feeling her soft hair in my hands as I cut near the base of her neck. With the final snip of the scissors, we placed her long braid in a a plastic bag, saving some of the strawberry-blonde hair as a keepsake for the girls. I had never seen Sarah with hair that short before. A memory from high school flashed through my mind. At fifteen, she was the most beautiful girl I had ever met. The first time I hugged her, I remember how her fragrant her hair was from her shampoo. Memories like that stay with you forever. We had our whole lives ahead of us then. Now, everything was completely different. We didn't know how much time was left, but we had hope. Sarah eyed the clippers on the table and I could sense she was a little nervous.

"Hey, Stone," I said to her. "You are so beautiful. Nothing will change that." I leaned in and kissed her.

"I know," she said. "I just want to help someone. Let's do this."

I turned on the clippers and held them buzzing in my hand for a moment. *Am I actually going to do this? This is crazy!* So many thoughts were going through my head. I started to shake. I didn't want to hurt her. With each pass of the clippers, her red hair fell like snow. She was gorgeous even with a buzz cut.

When the kids first saw Sarah at home with her new 'do, Maddie—being the kind-hearted soul that she is—whispered, "Mommy, you're so pretty. I love you." Kids are very straight to the point and we didn't know how they would react. I was so relieved that it didn't scare them or make them feel uncomfortable. When loved one, especially a parent, is sick, it can be confusing for kids. Sarah and I tried to help them adjust to what was going on, without telling them more than they needed to know.

Our chemo dates were every Friday. We looked at them as kid-free dates together where we could talk and laugh while she sat for hours. Every Friday morning, they accessed her port and ran blood tests, so there was a two-hour wait before each treatment would begin. To pass time, we'd sit in the hospital's bamboo garden. The sunlight would beam off her beautiful face and I'd just stare at her, taking mental pictures.

I wasn't dumb and neither was she; we both knew what was coming. We both knew things were about to get hard and that her body would weaken

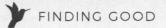

from the side effects of chemo. But we focused on living instead. She was dying. We both sensed it. But why waste the precious time we had left?

Every time Sarah felt good, we made memories. We even started a Facebook page called "Life Challenges and the Power of Positivity" where we would post photos and videos updating everyone on our journey. Every day, we vowed to make positive memories for the kids. She didn't look sick for the longest time. She was always smiling. Sarah had an entire palliative team at the hospital that loved her; oncologists and nurses who asked how she was and she would always check in and ask them how they were. Sarah was selfless that way. Everyone saw it and was inspired by it. She helped others find their good—even in her hardest times.

CHAPTER FIVE

Sarah - May 4, 2016 (Unedited video from Facebook)

I started chemo and have now had six chemo sessions and I have at least six more to go and it looks like the tumors are shrinking. I don't know how much they're shrinking but they're shrinking that's all that matters. My symptoms are not that bad and I am very lucky. When I was first diagnosed everyone kept telling me over and over, "You're so young," and now that I try to chemo I realized that that is a good thing. It's my silver lining chemo might be something that I'm doing but it's not me and it's not my whole story. I may be weak and I might be tired for a couple of days but I'm getting up and I'm living my life.

I was so sick before that I feel like I could run the world now. I feel so much better that even on my worst days of chemo, the days where I can't get out of bed and I'm nauseous I'm running in and out of the bathroom, it's still better because I have a good relationship with food again. I can sit outside and watch my kids play and I'm going to the girls' meeting tonight. I'm getting my son on the bus to go to preschool. These are things that before I was diagnosed I couldn't do. I was laying on my couch in tears.

I'm so thankful... the doctor said I have a palliative care team and they worry about just my symptoms. They said, "You know, if you're going for this entire process and we can only help you do one or two things, what is it that you want to do?"

I said, "I don't want to just do one of two things I want to be a mom and that's being a million things all at one time. And you know what? They've helped me be a mom. I'm very well medicated and I've learned to regulate all that and I'm able to be a mom again and that alone is that's all I wanted.

So, long story short, 2015 was by far the best and worst year of my life but 2016 is here. I'm stronger than ever; I'm really great and cancer will not divide me at all. It's just a little part of who I am and what I do. I'm a mom, a daughter, a wife, a sister, an aunt, a friend, a US Navy spouse. I am all of these things and cancer is just a little part of that, so I may have a year left, I may have ten years, I may have sixty years, but I know that I'm not living my life in fear. I'm getting up every day and I'm living my life the same way I would if I were helping. I'm not letting it hold me back and if cancer's done anything, it's made me appreciate life and finding the joy in every day.

Sarah - May 18th, 2016 (Unedited post from Facebook)

I've never been so terrified and eager at the same time. I'm choosing to fight hard and I want to live!! This surgery gives me the best odds and I'm up for the challenge. I can only be this way because I have a wonderful husband by my side encouraging me. Thank you, Johnathon, for everything you do. You're my rock and my best friend.

Sarah - June, 2016 (Unedited video from Facebook)

Johnny's way of coping with this illness is to stay positive. Sometimes it's hard and I'm scared—not that I'm going to die, but I'm scared of leaving a life unlived. I just want to make the most of it that I can. It's hard being on chemo but it could be so much worse. I'm so thankful that I can be at home. I'm scared that even with surgery I won't have much time. Appendix cancer is so rare and there isn't that much research on it.

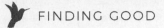

Last weekend, Johnny took the three girls to the father-daughter dance and they looked beautiful. They look forward to it and we're so lucky that the military housing that we live in puts the father-daughter dance on each year. It's a wonderful event and it's magical for the girls. I'm so glad they got to go; it was so fun and they were beautiful.

In between getting them ready and curling their hair and letting them pick out their favorite lip gloss to wear, the thoughts that are going through my mind are: *Will I feel good enough next year to do their hair? How many more father-daughter dances am I going to be able to help them pick out the right dress for and make sure they have the right shoes?* These are the thoughts that go through my mind on a daily basis.

It's really easy to only put the good out there because the good is ninety percent of our day; the bad is ten percent and it's hard and it's a battle. It's an inner battle that I have with myself on a daily basis. I wake up in the morning and I could take the easy route and I could cry and I could complain and I could say, "why me?"

I would love to do nothing but cry all day because that be easy, but I tell you, every day I wake up and I put a smile on my face and I focus on the blessings in my life. Because other than this horrible disease, my life is pretty great. I have a great husband and great kids and great support system and friends. It's not healthy to suppress the thoughts that I have, so I definitely process them. I say, "You know, man, this really sucks." I wonder this, I wonder that...

But more than anything, I remember that my children still need a very involved and active mother; my husband still needs a caring and kind wife. I do process these feelings and I go on about my day and I choose to put a smile on my face and to look at the bright side of things. The biggest takeaway that I want people to understand is that this is a marathon it's not a sprint. I don't expect to be cancer-free ever in my life. I don't want you to feel sorry for me. I just want to be real and I want to be realistic and show you that you know it's possible to have those moments and still have good days and a good life.

Johnny

After nine rounds of chemo, Sarah developed a bad cough that leads to throwing up. She reached a point where she couldn't lay flat. She was in a state of total suffering. Every night, I would put my hand on her chest to make sure she was still breathing. We had oxygen tanks in the house. It got to the point where she was throwing up several times a day.

The doctors and I were on a texting relationship by then I knew her entire medication schedule and would make sure she got everything she needed down to the minute. We were synced up and she would encourage me when I started to waiver. I felt like I was a registered nurse.

According to the MedStar Georgetown Cancer Institute, appendix cancer is rare and only affects 1,000 people in the United States each year. Tumors are either benign (non-cancerous) or malignant (cancerous). In many of these cases, common symptoms such as abdominal pain, increased abdominal girth, bloating, hernia, ovarian cysts or tumors in women, infertility, and ascites are misunderstood for years. One of the greatest challenges with appendix cancer continues to be correct and timely diagnosis along with access to the "Standard of Care" treatment now available to treat this disease which is cytoreductive surgery plus hyperthermic intraperitoneal chemotherapy (CRS/HIPEC).

When patients are misdiagnosed, they are less likely to benefit from CRS/HIPEC, and even with proper diagnosis many patients are never even offered it. This treatment, unavailable to patient population only a generation ago, has turned what used to be an almost certain death sentence into hope for thousands of patients around the world.

Unfortunately, by the time they found it in Sarah, it had already spread all throughout her stomach and to her bones. With that said, our only choice was to focus on the good every single day and live life to the fullest, right up until the end.

I hold Sarah's funeral back in Clinton, Illinois on November 10th, 2016. Her funeral is exactly as she wanted it to be, and the family buries her in Oak Park Cemetery—in a double plot with a couple's headstone.

The kids stuck together like a team. Some nights they even crawled into bed together when they were upset. The funeral for Sarah in Illinois is an emotional time for our entire family. Jackson was too young to know what had happened, but he sensed something was off. The twins would come up to me a lot and ask, "Why did mommy die? "How come we don't die, too, so we can be with mommy in Heaven, because Heaven is awesome."

"It doesn't work that way," I always replied. "If we die now, we won't get to see mommy." The kids know that God is love. Love is what got us through; keeping them around positive people made a big difference in how they coped with losing their mother.

In the months after Sarah's funeral, Allie uses her mom as an excuse to get into trouble; nothing major, just the typical kid behavior. I have to explain to her that her behavior isn't ok and that using her mommy as a reason to act out isn't acceptable. I let her know that we can talk about her mom whenever and as much as she wanted, but she still needed to learn responsibility for her actions.

Alyssa is a lot like me—more reserved, in control, and just gets stuff done. She plows through every problem. I have to check on her a lot to make sure she is okay and to get her to emotionally open up to me. Sometimes Alyssa would come crying to me and say, "Daddy, I miss Mommy so much."

"Mommy is in heaven looking down on us. She is watching you and protecting you. We've got this, we're a team. We will get through it together," I said. Allie wears her emotions on her sleeve. Maddie would cry every once in a while, too. They know how short life is. They are also scared of getting sick.

"Is cancer making me sick?" Maddie asked one night. "Will I die like Mommy?"

I tucked her into bed and said, "No, Maddie; you just have a cold. You will be better soon. You are very healthy and Mommy is your angel."

And it's true—Sarah really is watching out for us. One day when we returned home, I sat alone outside. The kids are off playing in the cul-de-sac and I take a moment to enjoy the peace and quiet. I miss Sarah more than

I can describe and it comes in waves. Some days, I feel confident as a single dad. I learn to cook (with a few casserole fails) and I coordinate our school and work schedules down to the minute. Other days, I feel overwhelmed and lost. As I sat outside, I could feel another wave of grief coming. That's the thing about grief, it ebbs and flows like the ocean.

I miss you, Stone...so much.

Then, a quiet hum came out of nowhere. A few feet in front of me, a bright, blue-green hummingbird appeared in midair. It fluttered as if to catch my attention.

I know it was a sign from Sarah. She was telling me that she heard me. From this that day on, hummingbirds appear regularly. Eventually, I learn the hummingbird is a symbol of courage and joy...which seems so perfect. Sarah was known for her ability to turn any bad situation into a good one. She was an inspiration to everyone she had contact with. No matter what she had going on personally, she always made it a point to put everyone else first.

Sarah will always be remembered for the fight she put up against cancer and her ability to stay positive throughout the entire journey. She was without a doubt one of a kind and has had direct impact on thousands of people. I am so lucky to have called her my wife and best friend.

Marriage is about being there for each other in sickness and in health—there was no way I was ever going to let her or the kids down. Up to that point, all the challenges we had as a couple and a family paled in comparison.

True love does exist; it's extremely powerful when you work together, but it's not just about a marriage. True love exists when you are there in faith for your friends, family, and people in your community. True love starts with finding the good in yourself and helping others discover it, too.

CHAPTER SIX

If you can't find your good, create it.

Considering everything that has happened, life is still beautiful. You have to be open to the signs from the universe. Life will throw things at you every single day and it's easy to get distracted. But you always have a decision: how are you going to react? Life will throw left hooks. There's always an outside force trying to influence your experience. It can make or break you.

Losing Sarah could have left me curled up in a ball, crying, and feeling broken. But I have a promise to Sarah that I would get up each day and live for our kids and for myself.

I am committed to keeping Sarah's name alive, and that means getting more involved with the local community. I am involved with the American Cancer Society, the Angels Family Foster Network, I Love A Clean San Diego, and several other organizations. As a natural leader, I always look for more ways to grow and serve the people around me.

In 2017, a neighbor suggests that I check out an event called Unleash the Power Within by Tony Robbins, an international speaker and life coach. My neighbor is a platinum-level member with Tony Robbins, which means she attends many of his events and even gets to travel with him. UPW seems like the perfect fit! I can attend a large seminar, receive the mindset and leadership training, and make tons of helpful contacts. However, the cost is out of my price range as a single dad, and I am trying to make ends meet with daycare and a nanny. My neighbor knows I am disappointed, but I have faith that another opportunity will come. A few days later, I receive an email from a Tony Robbins staff member informing me that I am being invited by Tony himself as a personal guest to the event and that I won't have to pay to attend!

On March 23, 2017, I head to Los Angeles to attend UPW live with 9,000 other people—including celebrities, public figures, and millionaires. I walk up to the VIP section near the stage and feel a little intimidated. Here I am, a farm boy from Illinois, hanging out with celebrities! Talk about a trip! Because I feel a little shy, I want to pick the corner seat in the back row. But then I start thinking there is was a reason why I am here. The universe works in mysterious and amazing ways, and I know that I am here to inspire someone else. I pick a seat in the middle so that others are around me.

The arena fills with a rush of motivated people and the energy is palpable. Tony takes the stage as the momentum builds and has us all cheering and high-fiving each other. At one point, he asks us to do an exercise where we turn to a neighbor and share a story for three minutes. I turn to my left and greet the man next to me. I share a story of sailor who marries his high school sweet heart and loses her to cancer.

"Where can I get this book?" he asks.

"Well, it's about me," I reply.

"It's a true story?"

"Yes," I say. "I'm that sailor and my wife Sarah passed away last November."

"You need to write this. People will be so inspired," he says.

I have never written a book before and it wasn't something I have considered before. So, I tuck the idea back in my mind and continue connecting with the amazing people around me. By Day 3, I have met so many diverse people who are all striving to make a difference in the world and become a better version of themselves. The best part is how I help

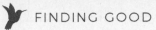

others begin this shift. For example, I give some words of encouragement to a woman who is a former athlete in the Russian Olympics. She is crying as she tells me how her father always called her stupid. I put my hand on her back and give her a pat for encouragement.

"First of all, you're here, in the VIP section of Tony Robbins' UPW," I say. "Think of how amazing this is. We all have a story; use all the negative energy from your past for something good. You can accomplish anything."

In this moment, I think about my story and the man who told me I need to write a book. I realize I need to have faith and do what seems to be almost impossible. I decide to take my own words to heart and ask others how they've created their books.

By the last day of UPW, I am open to a whole new world of possibility for myself and wanted to explore different ways of keeping Sarah's memory alive. After getting some helpful advice, I hire an editor and decided to move forward on writing the book...which is the book you are holding in your hand. *Life is incredible.*

I partner with Angels Foster Family Network to speak at their annual fundraiser on The US Grant Hotel in San Diego in May of 2017. I walk on stage in a fancy, 1920's-themed ballroom with champagne flowing and women dressed like flappers. It is the most important public speech I have ever done at the time and I don't want to blow it. I approach the microphone without any notes and just wing it. I remember to speak from the heart and share the Team Stone story and how Sarah wants to help people even after her death. It feels like I only talk for seconds and the rush of adrenaline takes me deep into the story. The memories of our family's journey flash in my mind and I know that I am here to be a catalyst and inspire others to do good in the world. Sarah is helping me create change from heaven.

By the time I am done, guests are da bbing their eyes with napkins and I receive a standing ovation from an audience of over six hundred people. When donations start, one man says, "I didn't intend to donate this much, but I am so moved by what Johnny has said." And it gets better...

The Grant family, who owns the hotel, offers to match whatever is donated.

We raise over $400,000 for the Expanding Caring Families Program!

On Mother's Day in 2017, I take the kids to Moore's Cancer Center and we plant a peach tree in her honor. Out of Sarah's death, new life is coming—literally and figuratively.

Thank you for guiding me, Sarah, I think to myself. *I'm not going to let you down.*

I continue working on the book and speaking to others in the greater San Diego area about finding good in every day. With each group I connect with, I feel our mission building. The media begins interviewing me about our story and I know that this is the beginning of something pretty incredible.

When Sarah was alive, one thing she always talked about was collecting backpacks and putting together little starter bags for foster kids. I connect with a few people who want to help me create a non-profit in Sarah's honor and finally make her vision a reality. In summer of 2017, I launch Simply Finding the Good, a non-profit dedicated to helping children entering the foster care system by providing them with things they need so they know they are loved and not alone.

Each year, approximately 400,000 children, like our son Jackson, enter the foster care system. The majority of the time they are removed from their home with only the clothes on their back. Going into the foster care system is an uncertain and scary time. We want these children to know they are loved and not alone by providing them with something they can call their own as they navigate through this difficult experience: a duffel bag filled with a pillow, blanket, books, journal, clothes, toys, stuffed animals, personal care items, and more.

Simply Finding the Good assembles their first care bags and delivers them. I bring the girls with me so they can see the importance of giving back to their community. It is amazing to bring the girls along and make them a part of their mom's dream.

We launch the non-profit's website and even brand it using a hummingbird in Sarah's honor. What I've realized is that her death isn't in vain. Because of her, I have been able to help so many people.

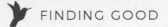

Now, it's your turn...

I want to remind you of just how precious life is. Keep living and moving forward. Be happy. Life is short and you get one shot. You have to spend your time creating a life that you truly want and deserve. If you want something, go make it happen. You have to step on the other side of fear. Once you get over that wall of fear, you may fall on your face, but get up and keep moving. You have to commit and keep going. A lot of people make the decision to change but then fall down and settle for a life that doesn't make them happy.

The world isn't as bad as the media and people make it out to be. There are so many positive people who want to help and who are helping every day.

I know, because I am one of them. I am so committed to living and spreading hope. I'm a small town farm kid with a story and a reason to live.

If I can do this, so can you.

If you don't appreciate what you have now, you won't appreciate anything in the future. Have gratitude for what you have now, even the smallest thing. There will be people and things that will try to block you, but you can't allow that to stop you. The unknown is where all the magic happens.

Life is short, live it.
Love is rare, grab it.
Anger is bad, dump it.
Fear is awful, face it.
Memories are sweet, cherish them.

- JOHNNY

30 DAYS TO FIND YOUR GOOD

Use the following pass downs to start your day with a momentum-building mindset. Keep a daily journal with your reflections and answers. After 30 days, you'll notice how your life is changing for the better...

DAY ONE

Life is always going to throw you curve balls, but it's how you see the problems that's going to make or break the situation.

The way you see life is the way it's going to be, so focus on the good and paint that beautiful picture called life.

How do you see life today?

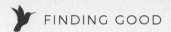

Finding Good
Daily Journal Reflection

_____

_____

_____

_____

_____

_____

_____

_____

_____

_____

_____

_____

_____

_____

_____

_____

_____

_____

_____

_____

DAY TWO

What if while learning to walk we never stood up and tried again?
We'd be crawling around through life never living to our full potential.

At what point did we stop getting up?

Why as adults do we let the fear of falling scare us into a life of settling
and unhappiness?

Today, simply go for it!

If you fall, get back up until you're running sprints!

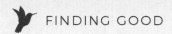

Finding Good
Daily Journal Reflection

_____

_____

_____

_____

_____

_____

_____

_____

_____

_____

_____

_____

_____

_____

_____

_____

_____

_____

_____

_____

_____

DAY THREE

Dig deep and remember what your favorite failure is.

What's that one big thing that happened, that at the time you couldn't believe you did or happened to you and now you thank God it happened?

How did you grow from it? Why is if now a blessing?

Remember everything happens for a reason, both good and bad.

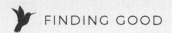

Finding Good
Daily Journal Reflection

_____

_____

_____

_____

_____

_____

_____

_____

_____

_____

_____

_____

_____

_____

_____

_____

_____

_____

_____

_____

DAY FOUR

Reach out to at least 3 people that are currently doing what it is you've always wanted to do: famous renowned authors, business owners, leaders... whatever it is you're trying to do or be.

Remember, they're no different than you.

We're all humans and we all have a story.

The only difference is they went for it...

Will you?

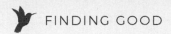

Finding Good
Daily Journal Reflection

DAY FIVE

Our mind is the most powerful tool we have. You have to start using it for you instead of against you.

Imagine you woke up with a brand new set of eyes this morning... a set of eyes that can only see the good in the problems at hand.

What is the good in today?

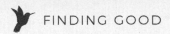

Finding Good
Daily Journal Reflection

DAY SIX

Life's way too short to hold yourself back!

Count your blessings and then leap on to the other side of fear and let your mind work for you instead of against you.

What are your blessings today?

Write down 3 things you're grateful for.

Watch your life instantly start making a turn for the better.

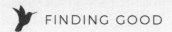

Finding Good
Daily Journal Reflection

DAY SEVEN

Remember, none of us are perfect and it's okay to be down sometimes. On days when you're really struggling, don't be afraid to ask for help. It's a lot easier to climb out of a deep hole when you have someone pulling you up.

Be patient and don't quit.
Your blast off is coming.

No matter how slow you're going, you're still going to be running laps around the people who haven't started yet. Remember to follow the signs that God gives us and trust that little voice telling you not to stop!

What are the signs?

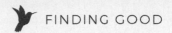

Finding Good
Daily Journal Reflection

DAY EIGHT

All the things that have happened in your past are not what's
holding you back...

You are holding yourself back.

You can't move forward while looking backwards! Focus on your "why"
and stop preventing yourself from creating the life you are destined to live.

What is your why?

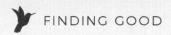

Finding Good
Daily Journal Reflection

_____

_____

_____

_____

_____

_____

_____

_____

_____

_____

_____

_____

_____

_____

_____

_____

_____

_____

_____

_____

DAY NINE

There will always be haters, struggles, worries, heartache, sadness and so many other factors in life, but I promise if you look hard enough there will always be something good.

Keep on your God-given path and remember, you only have one shot at life, so make it count.

Now go find your smile and never quit.

What makes you smile?

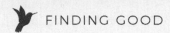

Finding Good
Daily Journal Reflection

DAY TEN

Say it, believe it, and it will happen.

I don't think people realize just how powerful our minds are. You can either pull yourself up or push yourself down with your very own thoughts.

Repeat after me: *No matter what life throws my way, I will never stop chasing my dreams. It's not over and I AM unstoppable!*

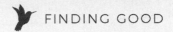

Finding Good
Daily Journal Reflection

DAY ELEVEN

You can't always control what happens to you, but you can ALWAYS control how you respond.

Every human on this planet has the same 24 hours in a day, so today when life tries to knock you down, choose to stand tall and focus on the solution/good...

At the end of the day, it's okay if you get knocked down but you cannot unpack and stay there.

How you can respond differently?

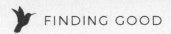

Finding Good
Daily Journal Reflection

_____

_____

_____

_____

_____

_____

_____

_____

_____

_____

_____

_____

_____

_____

_____

_____

_____

_____

_____

_____

_____

_____

DAY TWELVE

Treat negativity and hate like Medusa and don't even look at it. Instead, it's time to look at your life.

Life's too short and your time is too precious to be wasting it on anything less than living the way you are destined to live.

Do you accept it the way it is or do you want more?

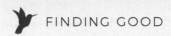

Finding Good
Daily Journal Reflection

_____

_____

_____

_____

_____

_____

_____

_____

_____

_____

_____

_____

_____

_____

_____

_____

_____

_____

_____

_____

DAY THIRTEEN

We all have that one defining memory that is currently holding us back from being the person we're meant to be.

Today, instead of using that memory as a moment of regret, use it to help someone that is currently going through what you once went through.

We all have a story. Once you start using it to help others, that memory will no longer hold you back.

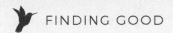

Finding Good
Daily Journal Reflection

DAY FOURTEEN

Take a walk outside and breathe. Notice the environment around you.

Find three things that your appreciate about the world around you.

Nature never worries, it just goes with the flow.

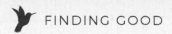

Finding Good
Daily Journal Reflection

DAY FIFTEEN

It's okay to be different in a world that spends 99% of the time focusing on negativity, hardships and struggles.

Be part of the 1% that focuses on the lessons, solution and beauty to this crazy thing we call life.

How can you be a one-percenter today?

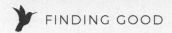

Finding Good
Daily Journal Reflection

_____

_____

_____

_____

_____

_____

_____

_____

_____

_____

_____

_____

_____

_____

_____

_____

_____

_____

_____

DAY SIXTEEN

Always trust your intuition.

That goes for your health, relationships, career and every other aspect of life. Intuition will appear as a gut feeling, an inner-knowing, or a confident voice inside your head that gives guidance on the next right step.

What is your intuition trying to tell you?

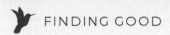

Finding Good
Daily Journal Reflection

DAY SEVENTEEN

Anybody can be good when times are good, but how good are you when times are bad?

Successful people know that success is all about focus, determination, and good habits.

If you are struggling in an area of your life, where can you get focused, increase your determination, and develop more discipline?

Every problem has a solution if you are willing to put in the effort to discover it. Respect yourself enough to go after a higher standard—one that you deserve.

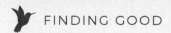

Finding Good
Daily Journal Reflection

DAY EIGHTEEN

You'll never be truly happy until you start appreciating the joys you already have.

Sit down for dinner as a family or with friends. Shut your phones off and go around the table saying what you're grateful for.

Not only will it bring you closer, it will also remind you just how beautiful your life already is.

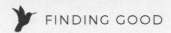

Finding Good
Daily Journal Reflection

DAY NINETEEN

Put your hand over your heart. Do you feel that? It's beating for a reason. You're an amazing person.

Remember, storms don't last forever. You will rise from the ashes like the Phoenix you truly are. Keep moving and you will fly high.

Can you dare yourself to dream bigger?

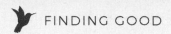

Finding Good
Daily Journal Reflection

DAY TWENTY

Set up a block of time every day dedicated to plugging away at your goals and growing.

No matter what you have going on, you have to make time for your goals. It's 100% impossible to get where you want to be in life if you don't make time for yourself.

Remember, people without out goals will always work for the ones who do. Use your 24 hours wisely.

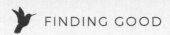

Finding Good
Daily Journal Reflection

_____
_____
_____
_____
_____
_____
_____
_____
_____
_____
_____
_____
_____
_____
_____
_____
_____
_____
_____

DAY TWENTY-ONE

Today, simply say yes.

If someone needs help, say yes.
If you receive a job opportunity, say yes.
If someone gives your something, say yes.

Try your very best to say yes before your brain convinces you to say no
like it's designed to do.

You have the power to control your mind.

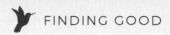

Finding Good
Daily Journal Reflection

DAY TWENTY-TWO

Negativity breeds more negativity.

What are you still angry about? Let it go.
What are you still sad about? Let it go.
What are you still scared of? Let it go.

When you let go, you let in the good.

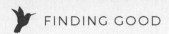

Finding Good
Daily Journal Reflection

_____

_____

_____

_____

_____

_____

_____

_____

_____

_____

_____

_____

_____

_____

_____

_____

_____

_____

_____

_____

DAY TWENTY-THREE

We all have special talents, skills, and abilities.

What are yours? List them out and then lift yourself up with positive thoughts.

You aren't here by mistake.

You are the key to unlock someone else's life.

Keep going and shining bright.

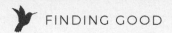

Finding Good
Daily Journal Reflection

DAY TWENTY-FOUR

Don't wait for the other shoe to drop.

It's easy to see the bad, fear the worst, and keep yourself in negativity.

How can you turn those thoughts around? Take 3 negatives and rewrite them as positives.

Flip the script; start filling your mind with positivity and that will help you find the good surrounding you.

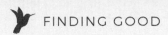

Finding Good
Daily Journal Reflection

DAY TWENTY-FIVE

Say thank you.

Who has helped you lately?

Give everyone the gratitude they deserve. The more you appreciate,
the more you receive.

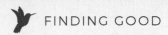

Finding Good
Daily Journal Reflection

_____

_____

_____

_____

_____

_____

_____

_____

_____

_____

_____

_____

_____

_____

_____

_____

_____

_____

_____

DAY TWENTY-SIX

Smile! Are you letting yourself be happy?

Go out into the world today and make eye contact and smile at 3 strangers.

You never know who you will impact with a small gesture of kindness.

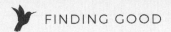

Finding Good
Daily Journal Reflection

DAY TWENTY-SEVEN

Take at least one picture of someone or something you love, that way you'll have that memory for the rest of your life.

If you can't find something in your day worthy of a picture, keep looking!

Your good is there, I promise.

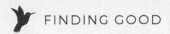

Finding Good
Daily Journal Reflection

DAY TWENTY-EIGHT

You will always receive what you give.

Be the reflection of what you'd like to see in the world.

How can you help someone today?

List 3 ways you can make a difference.

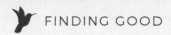

Finding Good
Daily Journal Reflection

DAY TWENTY-NINE

Write down 5 long-term and short-term goals.

Once you're done, hang them where you'll see them daily and start doing something towards conquering them every single day.

Remember, a person without goals will always work for the person with goals.

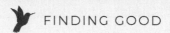

Finding Good
Daily Journal Reflection

DAY THIRTY

**You are ready and able to do good things
in this world!**

What do you want to be remembered for?

*What are you willing to do to ensure you're living the life you're
destined to live?*

Now, go make it happen!

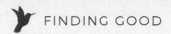

Finding Good
Daily Journal Reflection

_____

_____

_____

_____

_____

_____

_____

_____

_____

_____

_____

_____

_____

_____

_____

_____

_____

_____

_____

STONE

ABOUT JOHNATHON STONE

Johnathon Stone is a widower, Navy Chief, motivational speaker, life coach, and author who lives in southern California with his four children. He is the founder of Simply Finding the Good, a non-profit dedicated to serving children in the foster care system. His mission is to carry on a promise to his late wife, Sarah K. Stone, to help others live their best life through discovering the good in every day and spreading blessings to the world around them.

For information on his non-profit, visit SimplyFindingtheGood.com and to learn more about Johnathon, visit TeamStoneFindingGood.com.

Made in the USA
Middletown, DE
22 January 2020